Nutrient:

Food Groups And Diet

Crystal Reed

Table of content

Chapter 1

A Guide to the Importance of Nutrients for Optimal Health

Nutrients

Nutrients are substances that provide the body with the necessary materials to function properly and maintain good health. They are essential for growth, development, and the maintenance of various body functions.

Types of nutrients

They are two main types of nutrients:

Macronutrients

Micronutrients

Macronutrients

Macronutrients are nutrients that the body needs in large amounts to function properly.

There are three main types of macronutrients: carbohydrates, proteins, and fats.

Carbohydrates: these are an important source of energy for the body and can be found in a wide variety of foods, such as grains, fruits, vegetables, and legumes. Carbohydrates are classified as simple or complex based on their chemical structure and how quickly they are digested and absorbed by the body. Simple carbs, such as those found in sugar, candy, and soda, are quickly absorbed and can cause a rapid rise in blood sugar levels. Complex carbs, such as those found in whole grains, beans, and vegetables, are slower to digest and can help to maintain stable blood sugar levels.

Proteins: these are essential for the growth, repair, and maintenance of tissues in the body. They are made up of smaller units called amino acids, which can be obtained from both animal and plant sources. Animal sources of protein, such as meat, poultry, and dairy products, are considered complete proteins because they contain all of the essential amino acids the body needs. Plant sources of protein, such as beans, nuts, and grains, are considered incomplete proteins because they may not contain all of the essential amino acids.

Fats: these are an important source of energy for the body and are also necessary for the absorption of certain vitamins and minerals. Fats can be classified as saturated, monounsaturated, or polyunsaturated based on their chemical structure. Saturated fats, which are found in foods like meat, butter, and cheese, can increase LDL ("bad") cholesterol levels and increase the risk of heart disease. Monounsaturated and polyunsaturated fats, which are found in foods like nuts, seeds, and vegetable oils, can help to lower LDL cholesterol levels and reduce the risk of heart disease.

Micronutrients
Micronutrients are nutrients that the body needs in smaller amounts to function properly. These include vitamins and minerals.

Vitamins are essential for a wide range of functions in the body, including the metabolism of carbohydrates, fats, and proteins, the synthesis of hormones and neurotransmitters, and the maintenance of healthy skin, teeth, and bones.

Minerals are also essential for a wide range of functions in the body, including the formation of bones and teeth, the regulation of fluid balance, and the production of hormones and enzymes.

Benefits of Nutrients
There are many benefits to obtaining a variety of nutrients in your diet. Here are examples:

Protein helps to build and repair tissues, and is essential for the production of enzymes, hormones, and other molecules in the body.

Carbohydrates provide energy for the body, and are necessary for the proper functioning of the brain and nervous system.

Fats provide energy and help to absorb and transport fat-soluble vitamins. They also help to insulate the body and protect internal organs.

Vitamins and minerals are essential for a variety of functions in the body, including the immune system, metabolism, and the production of hormones and enzymes.

Water helps to maintain the body's balance of fluids, aids in digestion and metabolism, and helps to regulate body temperature.

Fibre helps to maintain bowel health and can help to lower cholesterol and blood sugar levels.

Calcium is important for the development and maintenance of healthy bones and teeth.

Iron is necessary for the production of red blood cells, which carry oxygen to the body's tissues.

Potassium helps to regulate heart function and water balance in the body.

Sodium helps to regulate blood pressure and maintain the body's electrolyte balance.

Zinc is important for immune system function and wound healing.

Vitamin A is important for eye health and the immune system.

Vitamin C helps to maintain healthy skin and connective tissue, and aids in the absorption of iron.

Vitamin D helps the body absorb calcium and is important for bone health.

Vitamin E is an antioxidant that helps to protect cells from damage.

Vitamin K is important for blood clotting and bone health.

Folate (vitamin B9) is necessary for the production of red blood cells and the synthesis of DNA.

Niacin (vitamin B3) helps to release energy from carbohydrates and is important for the functioning of the nervous and digestive systems.

Riboflavin (vitamin B2) is necessary for the metabolism of carbohydrates, proteins, and fats.

Thiamin (vitamin B1) is necessary for the metabolism of carbohydrates and the proper functioning of the nervous system.

Plant Nutrient Requirements:

Plants need certain nutrients in order to grow and thrive. These nutrients can be divided into two categories: macronutrients and micronutrients.

Macronutrients are nutrients that plants need in relatively large quantities and include:

Nitrogen (N): Nitrogen is an essential component of chlorophyll, the molecule that allows plants to convert light energy into chemical energy through photosynthesis. It is also a key component of proteins and nucleic acids. Nitrogen is often the most limiting nutrient for plant growth, so it is usually the first nutrient that plants will take up from the soil.

Phosphorus (P): Phosphorus is an essential component of nucleic acids, which are the building blocks of DNA and RNA. It is also a key component of ATP, the molecule that stores and releases energy in cells. Phosphorus is important for root growth and flower and fruit development.

Potassium (K): Potassium is an essential component of enzymes and plays a role in the regulation of water balance in plants. It is also important for the synthesis of proteins and carbohydrates. Potassium is necessary for strong stem growth and disease resistance.

Micronutrients are nutrients that plants need in small quantities but are still essential for plant growth and health. These include:

Iron (Fe): Iron is necessary for the synthesis of chlorophyll and the production of enzymes. It is also involved in the regulation of growth and development.
Zinc (Zn): Zinc is necessary for the synthesis of enzymes and hormones. It is also involved in the regulation of growth and development.
Manganese (Mn): Manganese is necessary for the synthesis of enzymes and hormones. It is also involved in the regulation of growth and development.
Plants can obtain these nutrients from the soil, through their roots. Some plants, such as legumes, have the ability to fix nitrogen from the atmosphere through a symbiotic relationship with nitrogen-fixing bacteria. In addition, plants can also obtain nutrients from fertilisers and other soil amendments.

It is important for gardeners and farmers to ensure that plants have access to the necessary nutrients in order to maximise growth and productivity. This can be achieved through the use of fertilisers or by maintaining the health of the soil through proper management techniques such as crop rotation and the addition of organic matter.

Chapter 2

The Major Classes Of Nutrients And Their Functions

Classes of nutrients:
Macronutrients:
Macronutrients are nutrients that our bodies need in large amounts. They include carbohydrates, proteins, fats and water.

Macronutrients provide calories (energy) to your body and fuel every cell in your body. These macronutrients come from foods like carbohydrates, fats and proteins. Carbohydrates can be found in fruits, vegetables or grains; proteins are found in meat or dairy products; fats come from oils or nuts.

Origin of carbohydrate:
Carbohydrates are found in grains (such as wheat and corn), starchy vegetables (like potatoes) and fruits.

Origin of fat:
Fats come from animal sources such as meat and dairy products or plant-based oils like olive oil or coconut oil.

Origin of protein
Protein comes from both animal sources (meat) and plant-based foods such as legumes (beans).

Micronutrients

A micronutrient is an essential nutrient that your body does not make and must get from other sources. Vitamins and minerals are two examples of micronutrients.

Vitamins:

Vitamins are organic compounds needed for the growth, development, and function of all cells in the body. They are usually absorbed through the diet but can also be made by bacteria that live in your intestines when you consume foods containing vitamin precursors (substances that release a single chemical unit).

Minerals:

Minerals are elements found in soil or water that affect our bodies' functions such as blood clotting, muscle contraction and enzyme activity.

Important of macronutrients:

Macronutrients are nutrients that the body needs in large amounts, and include carbohydrates, fats, fibre, minerals, protein and water. These macronutrients serve as the building blocks for our cells and are used to create energy.

Important of micronutrients:
Micronutrients are nutrients that the body needs in small amounts but play a critical role in maintaining good health. Vitamins and minerals fall into this category of micronutrients.

Why do we need carbohydrates, fats and proteins every day?

Carbohydrates, fats and proteins are macronutrients you need to eat every day. They're the building blocks of your diet and provide energy for your body to function.

Carbohydrates have a lot of different functions in the body. They're the main source of energy for most cells in our bodies, including our brain cells. Carbohydrates also help build muscle and support other bodily functions that are important for good health, such as digestion and hormone regulation (like insulin).

Fats also serve many important functions in the body—they help keep you warm when it's cold outside, cushion vital organs like your heart and spine so they don't get injured easily during movement or exercise, keep hair healthy by keeping moisture locked into the shafts without weighing down your locks with heavy products like gels or sprays...the list goes on! Fat is an essential nutrient that everyone needs in their diet because it provides certain vitamins (A & E) along with several minerals like iron which helps transport oxygen throughout our bloodstreams.

Conclusion

Whether you're trying to lose weight, gain muscle or just be healthier overall, knowing about the different types of nutrients is important. Macronutrients are nutrients that your body needs in large amounts—such as carbohydrates, fats, fibre and water. Micronutrients are essential nutrients that your body does not make and must get from other sources—like vitamins and minerals.

Chapter 3

A Comprehensive Guide to Vitamins and Their Benefits
Vitamins
Vitamins are essential nutrients that your body needs in small amounts to function properly. They are found in a variety of foods and are also available in supplement

form. There are 13 essential vitamins that your body needs:

Classification of vitamins
Vitamins are classified into two categories: fat-soluble and water-soluble.

Fat-soluble vitamins are stored in the body's fatty tissue and liver. These include vitamins A, D, E, and K. These vitamins can be stored in the body for long periods of time, so it is possible to have toxic levels if they are consumed in large amounts.

Water-soluble vitamins are not stored in the body and any excess is excreted in the urine. These include vitamins B and C. It is important to consume a consistent supply of these vitamins as the body does not store them.

Types Of Vitamins
Here is a list of the different types of vitamins and their functions:

Vitamin A: helps with vision and the immune system
Vitamin B1 (thiamin): helps with the metabolism of carbohydrates
Vitamin B2 (riboflavin): helps with energy production and the metabolism of carbohydrates, proteins, and fats
Vitamin B3 (niacin): helps with the metabolism of carbohydrates, proteins, and fats
Vitamin B5 (pantothenic acid): helps with the metabolism of carbohydrates, proteins, and fats
Vitamin B6 (pyridoxine): helps with the metabolism of proteins and carbohydrates and the production of red blood cells and neurotransmitters
Vitamin B7 (biotin): helps with the metabolism of carbohydrates, proteins, and fats
Vitamin B9 (folate): helps with the production of red blood cells and the metabolism of proteins and nucleic acids

Vitamin B12 (cobalamin): helps with the production of red blood cells and the proper functioning of the nervous system

Vitamin C: helps with the immune system and the production of collagen

Vitamin D: helps with bone health and the absorption of calcium

Vitamin E: helps with the immune system and the protection of cells from oxidative stress

Vitamin K: helps with blood clotting and the metabolism of proteins.

Some Important Parts of The Body Which Vitamin Plays A Vital Role

Vitamins for Eye Health:
There are several vitamins that are important for eye health, including:

Vitamin A: This vitamin helps to maintain the surface of the eye and is important for night vision. It can be found in foods such as carrots, sweet potatoes, and eggs.

Vitamin C: This vitamin helps to protect the eyes from oxidative stress and is important for maintaining the health of the blood vessels in the eyes. It can be found in foods such as oranges, strawberries, and broccoli.

Vitamin E: This vitamin helps to protect the cells in the eyes from oxidative stress and is important for maintaining healthy eyes. It can be found in foods such as almonds, sunflower seeds, and avocados.

Zinc: This mineral is important for maintaining the health of the retina and is found in high concentrations in the eye. It can be found in foods such as oysters, beef, and pumpkin seeds.

It is important to note that while these vitamins and minerals may be beneficial for eye health, it is generally best to get them from a balanced diet rather than through supplements. It is always a good idea to consult with a healthcare professional before taking any supplements.

Vitamins For Skin Health
There are several vitamins that are important for maintaining healthy skin. These include:

Vitamin A: This vitamin helps to maintain the integrity of the skin, and is necessary for the production of collagen, a protein that helps to keep the skin firm and elastic. Foods rich in vitamin A include sweet potatoes, carrots, and dark leafy greens.
Vitamin C: This vitamin helps to protect the skin from damage caused by free radicals, and is necessary for the production of collagen. Foods rich in vitamin C include oranges, strawberries, and peppers.
Vitamin E: This vitamin helps to protect the skin from damage caused by UV rays, and may also help to reduce the appearance of scars. Foods rich in vitamin E include nuts, seeds, and vegetable oils.

B vitamins: B vitamins, such as B12 and B6, are important for maintaining healthy skin. They help to keep the skin moist and may help to reduce the appearance of redness and inflammation. Foods rich in B vitamins include fish, poultry, and whole grains.

It is important to note that while vitamins can be beneficial for the skin, it is also important to maintain a healthy diet and lifestyle for overall skin health. This includes getting enough sleep, exercising regularly, and protecting your skin from the sun. If you are concerned about your skin health, it is always best to consult with a dermatologist or healthcare provider.

Vitamins For Hair Growth
There are several vitamins that are important for healthy hair growth. These include:

Vitamin A: This vitamin helps to produce sebum, a natural oil that helps to moisturise the scalp and hair.

Vitamin B: There are several types of vitamin B that are important for healthy hair, including B-12, B-6, and biotin (also known as vitamin B-7). These vitamins help to support the health of the hair shaft and scalp.

Vitamin C: This vitamin helps to promote collagen production, which is important for healthy hair growth.

Vitamin D: This vitamin helps to regulate the growth and cycle of hair follicles.

Vitamin E: This vitamin helps to moisturise the scalp and hair, and may also help to reduce inflammation.

It's important to note that while vitamins can play a role in healthy hair growth, a healthy diet and lifestyle are also important for maintaining healthy hair. In addition to getting enough of these vitamins through your diet or supplements, you can also use hair care products that contain these vitamins to help support healthy hair growth.

Vitamins for Immune System
There are several vitamins that are important for a healthy immune system. These include:

Vitamin A: This vitamin plays a role in immune function and helps to protect against infections. It can be found in foods such as sweet potatoes, carrots, and spinach.

Vitamin C: This vitamin is known for its immune-boosting properties and can help to reduce the severity and duration of colds and other infections. It can be found in foods such as oranges, strawberries, and kale.

Vitamin D: This vitamin helps to regulate the immune system and has been shown to play a role in the body's natural defence against infections. It can be found in fatty fish, egg yolks, and fortified foods such as milk and cereal.

It's important to note that while these vitamins may help to support a healthy immune system, they should not be used as a replacement for proper hygiene and medical care. If you are concerned about your immune health, it's always a good idea to speak with a healthcare professional.

Prenatal Vitamin List for Pregnant Women
During pregnancy, it is important for a woman to get sufficient amounts of certain vitamins to support the health of both the mother and the developing baby. Some of the vitamins and minerals that are particularly important for pregnant women include:

Folic acid: This B vitamin is important for the development of the neural tube, which eventually becomes the baby's brain and spinal cord. It is recommended that pregnant women take 400-800 mcg of folic acid daily.

Vitamin D: Vitamin D is important for the absorption of calcium and the development of the baby's bones and teeth. Pregnant women should aim for at least 600 IU of vitamin D per day.

Vitamin C: Vitamin C helps to support the immune system and is important for the production of collagen, which is a protein that helps to form the baby's skin, blood vessels, and connective tissue. Pregnant women should aim for at least 85 mg of vitamin C per day.

Vitamin B6: This B vitamin is important for the proper function of the immune system and the metabolism of carbohydrates and proteins. Pregnant women should aim for at least 1.9 mg of vitamin B6 per day.

It is generally recommended that pregnant women take a daily prenatal vitamin that contains these and other important nutrients. It is also important to eat a balanced diet that includes a variety of foods rich in these nutrients, such as leafy green vegetables, nuts, seeds, and fortified cereals.

Vitamins Memory Improvement
There is some evidence that certain vitamins may help with memory and cognitive function. However, it is important to note that taking supplements is generally not as effective as getting nutrients from a healthy diet.

Here are some vitamins that may be helpful for memory:

B vitamins: B vitamins, especially B6, B12, and folic acid, may help with memory and cognitive function. They can be found in foods such as poultry, fish, eggs, and leafy green vegetables.

Vitamin E: This vitamin may help to protect brain cells from oxidative stress, which can contribute to age-related cognitive decline. Good sources of vitamin E include nuts, seeds, and vegetable oils.

Vitamin D: Some research suggests that vitamin D may be important for brain function, including memory. Vitamin D can be synthesised by the body when the skin is exposed to sunlight, and it can also be found in foods such as fatty fish and fortified milk.

It is important to speak with a healthcare provider before starting any new supplement regimen, as some supplements can interact with medications or have other potential risks. Additionally, it is generally recommended to get nutrients from a well-balanced diet rather than relying on supplements.

Chapter 4

Definition Of Protein, Sources And Functions

PROTEIN:

Protein is a macronutrient needed in large amounts by the body for proper formation of cells into tissues and tissues into organs. Protein is the building blocks of body protein are organic molecules that are present in living organisms, they include many essential biological compounds such as hormones, enzymes and antibodies proteins consisting of amino acids, oxygen, nitrogen and sometimes Sulphur they are found in many foods. They are joined by peptide bonds. They are organ specific as the protein in the brain differs from muscle protein and liver protein but all in one organism. Protein molecules. Is larger than that of sugar molecules. The end products of protein are amino acids [the building blocks of the body].

CLASSIFICATION OF PROTEIN

Protein molecules are formed by one or more twisted and folded strands of amino acids. Amino acids are connected to each other by covalent bonds.

1.PRIMARY [1st level]: the structure of such protein is sequence of amino acids in a chain examples are haemoglobin [protein founds in red blood cell]

2. SECONDARY [secondary level]: the structure of such protein is formed by folding and twisting of the amino acids chain.

Examples are helix and the B pleated sheet. They are held in shapes by hydrogen bonds.

3. TERTIARY [3rd level]: such protein structures are formed by refolding and re -twisting of the secondary structure to form a larger three dimensional structure.

4. QUATERNARY [4th level]: this structure consists of more than one folded amino acid chain.

What are the food sources of protein?

 Meat- lean meats, beet, lamb, veal, pork.
  Poultry- turkey, chicken, duck games, goose.
  Fish and sea foods- crab, proms, fish, lobsters oysters, sanding, herrings, mackerels, catfish and crayfish.
Eggs.
Dairy products- milk, yoghurt, cheese, etc.
Almonds.
Seed.

Nuts, soya beans, peas, plant based protein often lack one or more essential amino acids while animal protein is of high biological value.

CLASSES OF AMINO ACIDS

Amino acids are classified into 3 groups: essential amino acids, non essential amino acids and conditional amino acids.

Essential amino acids: are the amino acids that cannot be made by the body therefore must be supplied and come from foods. The nine essential acids are isoleucine, Levine, lysine, methionine phenylalanine, threonine tryptophan and valine.

Non essential amino acid: these are amino acids that the body can produce, even if the diets are not rich in the amino acids these amino acids includes alanine, arginine, asparagine, aspartic acid, glutamic acids, glycine, praline, cysteine, serine and tyrosine the body cells can synthesise and obtained it in the body.

HOW MANY TYPES OF PROTEIN?

Proteins are of 2 types which are animal proteins and plant proteins. Animal proteins are proteins of high biological values with all the essentials amino acids present while plant proteins lacks one or more of essentials amino acids, but are high in fibre, phytochemicals and anti oxidative and anti inflammatory agent which gives it an advantage for health maintenance than animal proteins. Examples of plant protein are beans, lima beans, black eyed beans, bamboo nuts, seeds and nuts. Cereals such as Hungary, finger millet and rice have a certain amount of proteins. Examples of animal protein are meat such as beet, pork, veal, lamb poultry such as chicken, duck, turkey. Fish and sea foods such as sardine, catfish, herring, tilapia, mackerel, cry fish shrimps, crabs, periwinkles, oysters. Both types of proteins can be prepared and combined together in a meal to produce a high protein diet to manage a disease's condition.

Chapter 5

Definition Of Carbohydrates, Sources And Function
CARBOHYDRATE:

Carbohydrates are bio-molecules consisting of carbon (c), Hydrogen (H) and Oxygen (O) atoms with the ratio 2:1 just as in water. Carbohydrates perform numerous moles in living organisms, they are found in natural and processed foods. Carbohydrates refers to any food that is rich in the complex carbohydrate starch such as cereals, bread, and pasta or simple carbohydrates such as sugar found in candy, juices, and jams. It can also include chemical compounds such as acetic or lactic acid which are not normally considered as carbohydrates. Dietary fibre is carbohydrates but does not contribute to food energy (kilocalories) in humans but it is often included in the calculation of total nutrients taken by a person. Fibres are not digestible and absorbable. They only play a very vital role in the gastrointestinal tract system to control bowel movements.

SOURCES OF CARBOHYDRATE

Cereals and grains such as rice, corn, sorghum, Hungary rice (acha), finger millet (tamba) millet

Root & tubers such as yam, potatoes, water yam, cocoyam, sweet potatoes. Processed carbohydrates such as pasta (macaroni, noodles, spaghetti) carbonates sugary drinks such as colas, juices such as fruits juices and sweetened vegetables juices, jams syrups etc.

The body can break carbohydrates down into glucose. It helps in muscle contraction, It helps in temperature maintenance, regulating heartbeat and digestion of foods.

FUNCTIONS OF CARBOHYDRATE

1. Provides glucose as energy production.

2. It stored energy (glucose)

3. Building macromolecules

4. Assisting in lipid metabolism

5. Sparing protein (glucose synthesised from amino acids)

TYPES OF CARBOHYDRATE

Carbohydrates are classified into four types which are monosaccharides, disaccharides, oligosaccharides and polysaccharides.

Carbohydrates are formed by green plants during the process of photosynthesis from carbon dioxide and water.

MONOSACCHARIDE

Are simple sugars; they are the simplest carbohydrates that cannot be hydrolyzed into another simpler form. Examples of monosaccharides are glucose, fructose, galactose and mannose.

GLUCOSE:- Are naturally found in foods such as corn, root, cereals, honey, dried fruits, fruits juices, fresh fruits etc. These are healthy foods if consumed in moderation as part of an adequate diet. Glucose are considered natural sugars when consumed directly from whole foods such as dates.

FRUCTOSE:- Are sugar naturally found in fruits sweetest and more soluble than glucose? They are found in fruits such as apples, dates, pears, mangoes, oranges, and watermelon. Can also be found in some vegetables such as asparagus, mushroom, pepper. Fructose are crystalline monosaccharide.

GALACTOSE:- Are groups of simple sugar [monosaccharides] whose chemical formula is $C6H12O6$. It is usually found in nature combining with other sugars such as lactose, sugar found in milk galactose are less soluble and less sweet than glucose. Mammals that produce milk biosynthesize lactose from galactose and glucose. galactose are white, crystalline, water soluble hexose sugar. It is similar to glucose in structure but differs in the position of one hydroxyl group.

MANNOSE:- Is a group of monosaccharide that belongs to the groups of aldoses. Mannose occurs in microbes, plants and animals; free mannose is found in small amounts in some fruits such as oranges, apples, and also in mammalian plasma.

DISACCHARIDES

Disaccharides which is also called double sugar is the sugar formed by the combinations of two monosaccharides [simple sugar] they are soluble in water. The most common disaccharides are sucrose, lactose and maltose.

SUCROSE:- It is the most widely available and used disaccharides, commonly thought of as table sugar and naturally occurring sweetness. Is a sugar composed of glucose and fructose subunits produced naturally in plants and it's the main constituents of white sugar sucrose have the formula $C_{12}H_{22}O_{11}$.

LACTOSE: Is a disaccharides with the molecular formula $C_{12}H_{22}O_{11}$ is a sugar composed of galactose and glucose submits. Lactose comes from the lac meaning milk in Latin. Lactose is one of the components of milk which makes up to 2-8% of milk. Examples of lactose rich foods are milk, cheese, yoghurt, milk, chocolates, ice creams, butter etc. No lactose in fruits and vegetables.

MALTOSE:- Is a sugar of disaccharides consisting of two glucose units. Maltose is formed when starches like potatoes or rice are broken in the gastrointestinal tract system after digestion. It is then broken down into simpler sugar for energy. Maltose is obtained mostly from cooked foods. Maltose is a very important source of energy that can be stored or used immediately by the body after absorption. It has the formula $C_{12}H_{22}O_{11}$. The two units of glucose to form maltose are joined by an abound. Maltose is also referred to as malt sugar examples are cooked potatoes, rice, breakfast, cereals, bread, beer, cornmeal, wheat, barley, Hungary rice, sorghum finger millet.

POLYSACCHARIDES [COMPLEX CARBOHYDRATES]

Polysaccharides are long chains of monosaccharide [simple sugars] linked by glycosidic bonds; examples of polysaccharides are starch, glycogens and cellulose. They are made of molecules of smaller monosaccharide. Polysaccharide can be homopolysaccharide, in which all monosaccharides bond together are the same or a heterotopy saccharides where all monosaccharide binds together are different. Straight chains of monosaccharides are called linear polysaccharides while branch chains are called branched polysaccharides.

STARCH AND GLYCOGEN:- Glycogen and starch are produced by plants and animals. They are the most storage polysaccharides. Starch is a polysaccharides comprising glucose monomers. The simplest form of starch is the linear polysaccharides. Starch is the mixture of two polymers amylase and amylopectin. 10 – 30% amylase and 70 – 90% amylopectin are found in natural starch. It is the most important source of energy for humans. Starch are metabolised into glucose as energy so if there is excess glucose it stored in the liver as glycogen examples of starch are cereals, seeds, tubers [potatoes, yam, cocoyam cassava] roots, [carrots] and some fruits [green banana] plantains.

GLYCOGEN: Is a substance deposited in the body tissues in the form of carbohydrates. Glycogen is a polysaccharides that forms glucose on hydrolysis. Glycogen is stored in liver and skeletal muscles and small amounts in the brain glycogen is an important energy store for the body for future use. Liver glycogen regulates blood sugar levels and homeostasis while muscle glycogen plays a role in contraction of skeletal muscle for all physical activities in the body. Glycogen as starch is a complex carbohydrates [polysaccharides] at store excess glucose it is also referred to as 'animal starch' the constituent of amylopectin in plant starch is similar to the composition and structure of the constituents of glycogen when the body needs energy glycogen is broken down into glucose with glucagon the process is called glycogenolysis.

CELLULOSE: Is a polysaccharides made of chairs of glucose that constitutes the part of the cell walls of a plant is an insoluble substance of plant cells walls and of vegetables. Fibres it is made up of linear chain of b[1-4] linked D glucose units cellulose provides straight and rigidity to plant cells the formula of cellulose is [C6H10O5] it is odourless and has no taste cellulose serves as the plants cytoskeleton.

OLIGOSACCHARIDES

The formation of two, three or more monosaccharides join together by O-glycosides bonds. In rare cases it gives up to ten units of simple sugar [monosaccharides]. A saccharides is the unit structure of carbohydrates; it is smaller than polysaccharides which consist of more than 10 saccharides units.

CLASSIFICATIONS OF OLIGOSACCHARIDES

TRISACCHARIDES: These are oligosaccharides that comprised of three monosaccharides

TETRASACCHARIDES: They are oligosaccharides that comprise four monosaccharides.

PENTASCCHARIDES: Comprised five monosaccharides units

ITEXASACCHARIDES: Contains seven monosaccharides units.

TETRASACCHARIDES: Comprised eight monosaccharides units

POLYSACCHARIDES: Have nine no saccharides units

DECASSACHARIDES: Contains ten monosaccharides units

Examples of oligosaccharides are sucrose lactose and maltose

Chapter 6

Boost Your Health With Calcium - All You Need to Know

Calcium
Calcium is a nutrient required by all living things, especially humans. It is the most abundant mineral in the body and is essential for bone health.

Humans need calcium to build and maintain strong bones, and 99% of the body's reliable sources of calcium are in bones and teeth. It is also necessary to maintain healthy communication between the brain and the rest of the body. Involved in muscle movement and cardiovascular function. Calcium is naturally present in varieties of diet and food manufacturers add it to certain products.Supplements are also available.

Along with calcium, you also need vitamin D. Vitamin D helps the body to absorb calcium. You can get vitamin D from fish oil, fortified dairy products, and sun exposure.

This article examines why the body needs calcium, foods high in calcium, what happens when the body doesn't have enough calcium, and the pros and cons of taking supplements.

Why Do We Need Calcium In Our Body?
Calcium plays many roles in which the body benefits from. These include:

Bone Health
About 99% of the body's calcium is found in bones and teeth. Calcium is important for

bone development, growth and maintenance.

Calcium aids bone development as children grow. Even after a person stops growing, calcium continues to help maintain bones, slowing the loss of bone density that is a natural part of the ageing process. Women who have already gone through menopause may lose bone density more quickly than men and younger people.You are at an increased risk of developing osteoporosis and your doctor may recommend a calcium supplement.

Muscle
Calcium helps in regulating muscle contraction. When nerves stimulate muscles, the body releases calcium. Calcium helps the proteins in your muscles to work in contraction.

When the body excretes calcium from the muscles, the muscles relax.

Heart health
Calcium plays a vital role in blood clotting. The solidification process is complex and consists of several steps. These contain various chemicals, including calcium. Calcium's role in muscle function includes the maintenance of myocardial function. Calcium settled the smooth muscle that covers blood vessels. Various studies point to a possible association between high calcium consumption and low blood pressure.
Vitamin D is also important for bone health and helps the body absorb calcium.Learn more about vitamin D and why you need it.

Calcium is a cofactor for many enzymes. Without calcium, several important enzymes cannot work efficiently.

Studies also show that getting enough calcium can result in:

Reduced risk of developing hypertensive disorders during pregnancy
low blood pressure in adolescents
Lower blood pressure in those whose mothers had adequate calcium intake during pregnancy
Improved cholesterol levels
Reduced risk of colorectal adenoma, a type of benign tumour

List Of Foods Rich In Calcium:
Yogurt
milk
Fortified milk substitutes such as soy milk
sardines and salmon
cheese
Tofu
Green leafy vegetables such as broccoli, beet leaves, watercress, and kale
Lots of fortified breakfast cereals
fortified fruit juice
Nuts, especially almonds, sesame and chia
legumes and grains
cornmeal and corn tortillas

Dark green vegetables such as spinach contain calcium. However, it also contains a lot of oxalic acid. Studies have shown that oxalic acid reduces the body's ability to absorb calcium.

Deficiency Of Calcium
The following medical conditions or lifestyle habits can lead to low calcium levels, also known as hypocalcemia.

Binge eating, anorexia, and other eating disorders.
mercury exposure
overdose of magnesium
Long-term use of laxatives
Long-term use of some drugs, such as chemotherapy and corticosteroids
Chelation therapy for metal exposure
Deficiency of parathyroid hormone
People who eat a lot of protein and sodium can excrete calcium.
some cancer

Heavy consumption of caffeine, soda, or alcohol

conditions such as celiac disease, inflammatory bowel disease, Crohn's disease, and other gastrointestinal disorders

some surgical procedures, including removal of the stomach

kidney failure

pancreatitis

vitamin D deficiency

Phosphate deficiency

The body excretes some calcium in sweat, urine, and faeces. Foods and activities that promote these functions can lower calcium levels in the body.

Vitamin D Is Required For Calcium Absorption

Your body needs vitamin D to absorb calcium, which means that if you're deficient in vitamin D, you won't be able to fully benefit from a calcium-rich diet.

Vitamin D can be obtained from certain foods such as salmon, egg yolks and mushrooms.

Like calcium, vitamin D is added to some foods. For example, milk often contains vitamin D.

Sunlight is the best option for generating vitamin D. The skin produces vitamin D naturally when exposed to sunlight. Darker-skinned people also don't produce vitamin D, so supplements may be needed to avoid a deficiency.

Why Do Children Need Calcium?
You only have a chance to build strong bones when you are a child or teenager. Children who get enough calcium start adult life with the strongest possible bones. This helps prevent bone loss later in life.

Toddlers and infants need calcium and vitamin D to prevent a disease called rickets. Rickets softens bones, causing bow legs, underdevelopment and sometimes muscle pain and weakness.

Chapter 7

All About Folic Acid (Folate): Health Benefits and More

Folic Acid (folate)
The water-soluble natural vitamin B9 is known as folate, and it may be found in a variety of foods. In the form of folic acid, it is also added to meals and offered as a supplement; this form is actually more readily absorbed than that obtained from dietary sources (85% vs. 50%, respectively). Folate participates in protein metabolism and aids in the formation of DNA and RNA. It is essential for the breakdown of homocysteine, an amino acid that, in excessive concentrations, can have negative

effects on the body. Folate is essential during times of fast growth, such as during pregnancy and foetal development, and is also required to generate healthy red blood cells.

What Is Folic Acid (folate)
The man-made B vitamin folate is called folic acid. Natural sources of folate include several fruits, vegetables, and nuts. Vitamins and fortified foods include folic acid.

The nutrients folate and folic acid assist the body in producing healthy new red blood cells. Every region of your body receives oxygen thanks to red blood cells. Anaemia can occur if your body can not produce enough red blood cells. You become pale, exhausted, or weak when you have anaemia because your blood is unable to deliver enough oxygen to your body. Additionally, if you do not consume enough folic acid, you may develop folate-deficiency anaemia.

Why Do Women Need to Folate Most?
during and before pregnancy. Neural tube abnormalities, which are significant birth malformations, are prevented by folic acid in foetuses. These birth abnormalities frequently occur before a woman is aware that she is pregnant during the first few weeks of pregnancy. Additionally, folic acid may protect against various birth abnormalities including early miscarriage (miscarriage). Due to the fact that roughly 50% of pregnancies in the US and Africa (Nigeria) are unplanned, specialists advise all women to consume adequate folic acid, even if you are not attempting to conceive.

to maintain the health of the red blood cells by promoting their development. A condition known as folate-deficiency anaemia can result from a lack of folic acid. Women of reproductive age are more likely than men to have folate-deficiency anaemia.

How To Get Folic Acid?

There are two ways to get folic acid.

By The Meals You Consume. Spinach, almonds, and beans are a few examples of foods that naturally contain folate. Foods that have been fortified with folic acid are known as "enriched foods," and examples include breads, pastas, and cereals. If you want to know if a food includes extra folic acid, look for the word "enriched" in the ingredients list.

The Vitamin. The majority of multivitamins marketed in the US and Nigeria have 400 micrograms, or 100% of the RDA, of folic acid.

How Soon Should I Begin Consuming Folic Acid (Pregnant women)?
Within the first 3–4 weeks of pregnancy, birth abnormalities happen. Therefore, during those crucial early stages when your baby's brain and spinal cord are forming, it's crucial to have folate in your system.

When you were trying to get pregnant, your doctor likely advised you to start taking prenatal vitamins with folic acid. According to one study, women who took folic acid for at least a year before becoming pregnant reduced their risk of having an early delivery by 50% or more.

The CDC advises starting folic acid daily for at least a month before becoming pregnant and continuing it daily while you are pregnant. The CDC does advise all women of reproductive age to take folic acid daily, though. You may thus begin taking it even early.

When you get pregnant, take the prenatal vitamin you choose to your OB to make sure it has the necessary levels of all the nutrients you require, including folic acid. There are variations among prenatal vitamins, and some may include fewer or more of the vitamins and minerals you require.

What Dosage Of Folic Acid Should I Use?
All women of reproductive age should consume 400 mcg of folate every day. Verify that your daily multivitamin has the required quantity if you take one. You can use folic acid pills instead of a multivitamin if you don't want to for any reason.

The daily folic acid recommendation during pregnancy is as follows:

400 mcg while you're attempting to conceive
400 mcg during the first three months of pregnancy
Pregnancy months four through nine: 600 mcg
500 mcg when breast-feeding

Good Sources Of Folic Acid In Food
Dark-green leafy veggies like spinach
orange juice with oranges
Nuts\Beans

Meat

poultry (chicken, turkey, etc.)

whole grains

You may increase your folic acid intake with the following foods:

Breakfast cereals fortified with 400 mcg, or 100% of the DV 3/4 cup

Beef liver, cooked and braised, 3 oz., 215 mcg

179 mcg: cooked, boiling, ripe lentil seeds. 1/2 cup

115 mcg: frozen, cooked, and boiling spinach 1/2 cup

110 mcg: cooked, enhanced egg noodles 1/2 cup

Breakfast cereals fortified with 25% of the DV at 100 mcg 3/4 cup

Great Northern beans, cooked, 1/2 cup, 90 mcg

Can I Get Enough Folic Acid In Foods Alone?

Yes, a lot of individuals consume enough folic acid from diet alone. Several foods contain a lot of folic acid. For instance, each serving of many morning cereals has 400 micrograms of folic acid, which is 100% of the daily required intake. To be certain.

Some women, particularly those who could become pregnant, might not get enough folic acid through diet. Mexican Americans and African-American women are also more likely to not obtain enough folic acid every day. If you want to receive the 400 micrograms of folic acid you require each day, talk to your doctor or Dietitian about whether you should take a vitamin.

After Menopause, Do I Still Require Folic Acid?
Yes. After menopause, women still require 400 mcg of folic acid daily for optimal health. How much folic acid you require should be discussed with your doctor or Dietitian.

Neural Tube Defects
Birth problems called "neural tube defects" concern the brain and spinal cord's inadequate development. These are the most typical neural tube defects:

Anencephaly, a condition in which the skull, scalp, and brain do not develop properly, and encephalocele, in which brain tissue protrudes out to the skin via a hole in the skull, are examples of spina bifida.
These birth abnormalities occur within the first 28 days of pregnancy, frequently before the mother is even aware that she is expecting.

Because of this, it's crucial for all women of reproductive age to consume adequate folic acid, not just those who are attempting to conceive. Anyone who could get pregnant should be careful to acquire enough folic acid because half of pregnancies are unplanned.

Supplement Interactions With Folic Acid
The absorption or metabolism of folic acid by your body might be affected by a number of drugs.

These drugs include, as examples:

Sulfasalazine (Azulfidine), sulfamethoxazole/trimethoprim, and other anti-seizure drugs such phenytoin (Dilantin), carbamazepine (Tegretol), and gabapentin (Neurontin) (Bactrim)
Folic acid levels may be decreased by phenytoin. However, it's also believed that folic acid intake may reduce the effectiveness of phenytoin. If you're taking both, your doctor might need to change the dosage of phenytoin you're taking.

A drug called methotrexate stops your body from using folic acid. During therapy, you could be told to take a folic acid supplement if you're taking it for an autoimmune disorder. However, you can be told not to take folic acid if you're taking methotrexate for cancer.

Negative Effects Of Folic Acid Supplements
Up to 400 mcg of folic acid per day is typically regarded as safe. Additionally, this dose range is often well tolerated. High doses of folic acid are associated with the majority of its adverse effects (e.g., 15 mg daily).

These adverse consequences include, for instance:
reduced appetite
Nausea
Bloating
releasing gas
unpleasant aftertaste
sleeping issues
Consciousness issues
becoming agitated

Chapter 8

Vitamin A Deficiency: What You Need to Know

Vitamin A Deficiency

The absence of sufficient vitamin A in the body is known as vitamin A insufficiency. Vitamin A is a fat-soluble vitamin that is essential for numerous body processes, including cell proliferation, immune response, and eyesight. A lack of food intake or an issue with absorption can lead to a vitamin A deficit. It is a significant public health issue, especially in underdeveloped nations where it is the main contributor to infant avoidable blindness.

Importance of Vitamin A

Maintaining clear vision, a strong immune system, and normal organ function all depend on vitamin A. Additionally, it contributes to the growth and maintenance of healthy mucous membranes and skin. Night blindness and an elevated risk of

infections are two conditions that can result from a vitamin A deficiency. Consuming foods like:
sweet potatoes
carrots
spinach
and eggs
can help you acquire the necessary amount of vitamin A in your diet.

Causes of Vitamin A Deficiency
Lack of dietary intake: Lack of food intake is the most frequent cause of vitamin A insufficiency. This can happen in communities who rely largely on a single staple meal that is deficient in vitamin A, such rice. This is especially common in low-income nations where fruits, vegetables, and sources of vitamin A derived from animals are frequently absent from the diet.

Malabsorption: The body's capacity to absorb vitamin A from diet can be impacted by several medical diseases, including

Crohn's disease and celiac disease. When the body has trouble absorbing and utilising nutrients from meals, they are ejected as a result of malabsorption..

Increased need: The demand for vitamin A may be higher in some groups, such as those who are pregnant or nursing, and a deficit may result from insufficient dietary consumption. A deficiency is also more likely to occur in people with chronic diseases like HIV/AIDS because their systems may need extra vitamin A to fight against infection.

Symptoms of Vitamin A Deficiency
Night blindness: Night blindness, or having trouble seeing in dim light, is one of the initial symptoms of vitamin A insufficiency. Degeneration of the retina, the area of the eye that detects light, is to blame for this.

Dry eyes and conjunctivitis: Dry eyes and conjunctivitis are additional symptoms of vitamin A insufficiency (inflammation of the conjunctiva, the clear membrane that covers the white part of the eye and the inside of the eyelids). The eyes may feel scratchy, burning, and uncomfortable as a result.

Dry skin and hair: People who are vitamin A deficient may have dryness and scaliness of the skin and hair. Additionally, the skin may thicken and become more prone to infection.

Increased susceptibility to infection: A vitamin A shortage can increase vulnerability to illnesses including measles, diarrhoea, and respiratory infections since vitamin A is essential for immune function.

Diagnosis of Vitamin A Deficiency
Physical examination: Symptoms of vitamin A insufficiency, such as dry skin or eyes, can be detected by a physical examination..

Blood test: The amount of vitamin A in the body may be determined via a blood test. A deficiency is indicated by low blood levels of vitamin A.

Treatment of Vitamin A Deficiency

Diet: The main method of treatment for deficiency is to increase consumption of foods high in vitamin A, such as liver, sweet potatoes, and leafy green vegetables. Other necessary minerals, such as beta-carotene, which the body transforms into vitamin A, are also abundant in these meals.

Supplements: If a person's diet does not provide them with enough vitamin A, they can purchase vitamin A supplements. There are several types of these supplements, including tablets, drops, and injections.

Fortification: In order to boost the population's total consumption of vitamin A, a public health intervention known as vitamin A fortification includes adding vitamin A to regularly consumed foods like wheat or oil. This is especially helpful in underdeveloped nations where there is limited availability to foods high in vitamin A.

Avoiding a vitamin A shortage

Through a mix of dietary and non-dietary measures, vitamin A deficiency can be prevented.

Vitamin A-rich foods including leafy green vegetables, sweet potatoes, carrots, squash, and fruits like papaya and cantaloupe are some examples of dietary strategies. Fish, liver, and fortified meals like milk and cereal can all help avoid deficiencies.
Non-dietary approaches include giving vitamin A supplements to vulnerable groups like young children and expectant mothers. The prevalence of vitamin A insufficiency has been successfully decreased in certain poor nations by widespread distribution initiatives for children.

Education and public awareness: Increasing knowledge of the value of vitamin A and how to consume it can also aid in preventing deficiency. This might involve educating people on the significance of eating a balanced diet and the dietary sources of vitamin A.

Access to health care: By recognizing and treating Vitamin A insufficiency early on, having access to routine health examinations and treatments, especially for individuals who are at high risk of deficiency, can help prevent deficiency.

By lowering the prevalence of viral disorders that might result in vitamin A malabsorption, better sanitation and hygiene can help prevent vitamin A insufficiency.